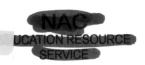

Ladybird's
Remarkable
Relaxation

by the same author

Frog's Breathtaking Speech
How Children (and Frogs) Can Use Yoga Breathing
to Deal with Anxiety, Anger and Tension
Michael Chissick
Illustrated by Sarah Peacock
ISBN 978 1 84819 091 7
eISBN 978 0 85701 074 2

of related interest

Six Healing Sounds with Lisa and Ted
Qigong for Children
Lisa Spillane
ISBN 978 1 84819 051 1
eISBN 978 0 85701 031 5

The Panicosaurus
Managing Anxiety in Children Including
Those with Asperger Syndrome
K.I. Al-Ghani
Illustrated by Haitham Al-Ghani
ISBN 978 1 84905 356 3
eISBN 978 0 85700 706 3

Ladybird's Remarkable Relaxation

How children (and frogs, dogs, flamingos and dragons) can use yoga relaxation to help deal with stress, grief, bullying and lack of confidence

MICHAEL CHISSICK

Illustrated by
SARAH PEACOCK

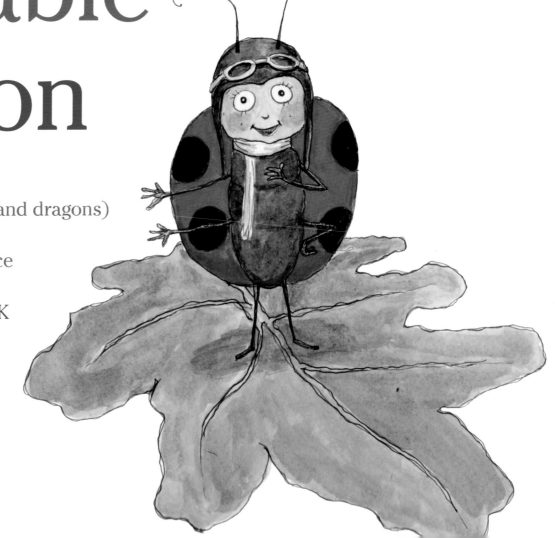

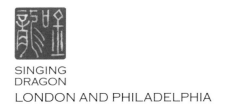

SINGING DRAGON

LONDON AND PHILADELPHIA

First published in 2014
by Singing Dragon
an imprint of Jessica Kingsley Publishers
73 Collier Street
London N1 9BE, UK
and
400 Market Street, Suite 400
Philadelphia, PA 19106, USA

www.singingdragon.com

Library of Congress Cataloging in Publication Data
Chissick, Michael.
  Ladybird's remarkable relaxation : how children (and frogs, dogs, flamingos and dragons) can use yoga
relaxation to help deal with stress, grief, bullying and lack of confidence / Michael Chissick ; illustrated
by Sarah Peacock.
     pages cm
  ISBN 978-1-84819-146-4 (alk. paper)
  1. Relaxation–Juvenile literature. 2. Hatha yoga–Juvenile literature. 3. Hatha yoga for children–
Juvenile literature. I. Peacock, Sarah, illustrator. II. Title.
  RA785.C454 2013
  613.7'046–dc23
                          2013009725

British Library Cataloguing in Publication Data
A CIP catalogue record for this book is available from the British Library

ISBN 978 1 84819 146 4
eISBN 978 0 85701 112 1

Printed and bound in China

This book is dedicated to:

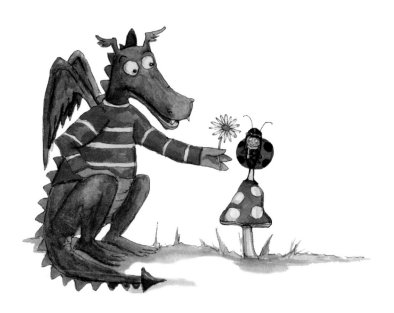

Amelie, my gorgeous little girl *SP*

David William Morris, a remarkable friend *MC*

Luke Watts (1999–2011), who loved Ladybird Relaxation *MC*

ACKNOWLEDGEMENTS

I would like to thank the head teachers who had the courage and belief to allow yoga in their schools as part of the integrated school day. Thanks to them, Ladybird Relaxation has grown and developed into an activity that has helped, and will continue to help, hundreds of children to deal with stressful aspects of their lives.

In particular, I would like to express my immense gratitude to:

Stewart Harris, Head of Phoenix School, Bow, East London.

Karen Scudamore and Nick Heald, Heads of Holdbrook Primary School, Waltham Cross, Hertfordshire.

Sarah Goldsmith, Head of Downfield Primary School, Cheshunt, Hertfordshire.

Lynda Pritchard, Head of Warren Primary School, Thurrock, Essex.

I would also like to say an enormous thank you to all the class teachers, teaching assistants and learning support assistants who I work with week in and week out. With a special mention for Anthony Olejnik at Holdbrook Primary, and the amazing staff at both Phoenix School in Bow and Woodcroft School in Loughton. Without all these people, Ladybird Relaxation would not fly.

Finally, thank you to all the children who regularly relax imagining the tiny Ladybird on its gentle journey.

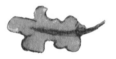

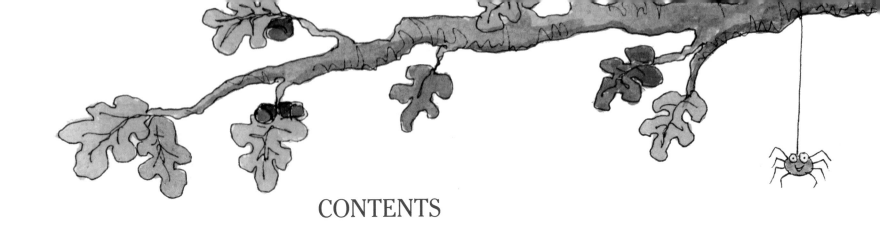

CONTENTS

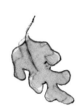

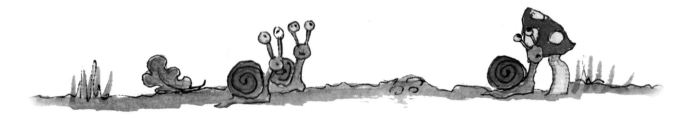

Guidance for Teachers and Parents

Introduction

Ladybird Relaxation has been the jewel in the crown of my yoga lessons since 1999, and is the most successful relaxation technique that I have ever used in my career as a children's yoga teacher. It is successful because:

- it is remarkably simple, fun and easy to learn

- everyone can do it

- once learnt, children can take it and use it anywhere

- it is genuinely yoga based

- it works! Children become relaxed.

Who is this book for?

Ladybird's Remarkable Relaxation is aimed at primary and elementary school teachers, head teachers, teaching assistants and people who work in the field of special needs who may have little or no knowledge of yoga, and is suitable for children of all ages.

It is also a *must* for children's yoga teachers and will save them hours of planning time.

This yoga story book is also for parents who are looking for a fun and engaging story to teach their children about coping with difficult emotions.

What are the benefits of relaxation for children?

There can be little argument that relaxation is beneficial for children, whether in school or at home. Based on anecdotal evidence alone it is clear that relaxation can help to:

- calm busy minds and young nervous systems; which in turn helps children to deal with anxiety and tension, and ultimately reduces stress

- relax muscles, joints and the whole body, as well as revitalising tired children (and teachers and parents too!).

More specifically, children can practise Ladybird Relaxation at times of stress anywhere, anytime, with immediate results.

Main goal

The main goal of Ladybird Relaxation is to give children a relaxation technique that, once learnt, they can use anywhere and anytime to help them to cope with a problem, without depending on anything or anyone but themselves. In other words, to give children the skills, knowledge and responsibility to manage their own relaxation.

Do children enjoy Ladybird Relaxation?

I am still amazed that even the most exuberant children enjoy this relaxation. The majority of children I teach are happy to lie still on their mats for around six minutes. They look forward to Ladybird Relaxation and complain if, for any reason, I have to leave it out; and they are forever telling me how they use relaxation outside of the yoga lesson.

Here are some examples of how Ladybird Relaxation has helped children:

CASE STUDY 1

Five Year 5 girls were sharing a room on their school trip to the Isle of Wight. For most of them it was their first time away from home without parents. The first night they talked and giggled and couldn't get to sleep. It was suggested that they try Ladybird Relaxation, which they did three times and then fell asleep.

CASE STUDY 2

It is easy to practise Ladybird Relaxation at the desk; which is exactly what a Year 6 teacher did with her class every morning before the SATS exams last year. She is adamant that her year group were calmer, more relaxed and better able to cope with the exam stress.

How can Ladybird help children deal with problems?

Having practised yoga and all things related since the 1970s my conclusion is that within each of us there is a vast reservoir of courage, wisdom and compassion that we can call upon in times of problem and crisis. From those three elements can grow:

- self-respect
- respect for others
- perseverance
- coping skills
- confidence
- self-awareness.

My whole approach to children's yoga has been developed with the aim to help children realise that they can tap into that reservoir in order to enhance their self-efficacy, self-belief and self-esteem.

Ladybird Relaxation has been central to reaching that reservoir. I believe that when children are relaxed they are most receptive to the idea that they have these inner resources; resources that can then colour their decisions and actions in a positive way.

Yoga speak

Ladybird Relaxation is based on the practice of yoga nidra. Yoga nidra is also called "rotation of consciousness," which, in the context of the technique described in this book, simply means directing your attention or focus to specific body parts in a specific order. Yoga nidra is seen in the yoga world as a "systematic method of inducing complete physical, mental and emotional relaxation." In fact, it is great practice for improving focus.

How to use this book

IN SCHOOL

The story can be easily integrated into your provision for self-esteem enhancement, for example SEAL, PSHE or Circle Time in the UK.

The story highlights four typical problems that children experience:

- inability to cope with workload

- being bullied

- lacking confidence

- grief.

Read the story to your class and invite them to talk about their own problematic situations, which may be similar to those that Frog and friends experience.

The next stage is to use the Ladybird Relaxation Script, which you will find on page 47. It is designed for whole-class participation either in the hall or at desks. In the hall is best. If possible let each child have their own mat or space. Have your resources (ladybird puppet, bells, ladybird on string) ready.

As you become more familiar and confident with the script feel free to adapt it to meet the needs of your children and what may be happening in front of you. For example, if a child is moving their hands when they are supposed to be keeping them still you could say: "If you can keep your hands still the ladybird may land on you."

Class teachers will be able to practise with the whole class immediately. It is safe, easy to use and fun. I have used this technique with children from nursery age to Year 6 (3 to 11 years old). It's tried, tested and *works*!

CHILDREN'S YOGA TEACHERS

I recommend that you dedicate 5–6 minutes to Ladybird Relaxation towards the end of your 30-minute lesson. Use the script on page 47 and read this guidance to enrich the experience.

PARENTS

Read the story with your child or children and practise together. Take turns to be the leader. Share examples of your own experiences where relaxation has helped you be in the right life state to find courage, wisdom and compassion to help with a problem. Of course deposit practice points in the "relaxation bank" by practising even when your child does not have a problem.

Motivating children to be still

Often, for the first 3–4 weeks after I have introduced this technique, I ask the children to think about how the tiny, shy ladybird may be feeling; that any movement may frighten or startle the ladybird, and to show me how kind they can be by being as still as they can. It's a motivation that works well. Try it!

VOICE

Your voice is the key. Use a strong, warm, calm voice. Too low and children can fall asleep or get bored because they cannot hear you. Too loud and harsh and you'll be wasting your time. Usually I teach in a school hall with the mats arranged in a circle. Some halls absorb sound easily so do some tests before you start.

STRUCTURE AND ROUTE

It is a vital aspect to this technique that the ladybird takes the same route each time. It can be clockwise or anti-clockwise. Rarely do I use the words *left* or *right* because that can be confusing for many children, preferring to use the words "the *other* shoulder, *other* thumb, *other* toe" instead. By keeping to the same structure each time you will reinforce the activity, which will help children learn to the point that they can practise this on their own anywhere.

BELLS

Ringing a bell or simple triangle each time the ladybird lands on a body part will help the children focus. At the end of the relaxation continuously strike the bell or triangle to signal that Ladybird Relaxation is finished. It's fun!

EXPECTATIONS

Do set your expectations at realistic levels. Some children will fidget to some degree – that is normal. You will find, though, that they are fidgeting a lot *less* than they normally do; and through regular practice fidgeting and most movement will disappear – so persevere!

Years 3 to 6 (8–11 years old) find it easier to be still, whereas Reception to Year 2 (4–7 years old) need more input from you. I will only teach to nursery classes (3–4 years old) when I think they are ready for it, which is normally by the summer term if I have been teaching them since September in that academic year.

SPECIAL EDUCATIONAL NEEDS CHILDREN

If you teach any special needs children, who may not be able to follow your verbal instructions or may find stillness a challenge, ask another adult to use a ladybird finger puppet with the child so they can feel it landing gently on the toe, knee and so on. I often use Ladybird Relaxation in special needs schools with the ladybird finger puppet suspended on a string.

LADYBIRD PUPPET ON A STRING

Another highly successful approach is to have a ladybird finger puppet on a length of string tied to a pole. Children will do *anything* to be the person controlling the pole – even improve their behaviour; and those on the floor or chairs who want to be landed on by the ladybird will try even harder to be still.

CREATE INDEPENDENCE

Encourage children from Year 3 to Year 6 (8–11 years old) to lead the Ladybird Relaxation. It's helpful to have ready a laminated A4 sheet listing the landing points. I normally choose two children: one to read from the sheet and the other to control the pole. I encourage readers to adlib with their own ideas. This works very well and there are lots of opportunities for shy children to address the class without fear of interruption.

BREATHING

I aim to include a simple breathing technique in the Ladybird Relaxation 3–4 weeks after the first session. This is because my initial goals are for the children to learn the technique, remember the sequence and become able to use it independently. Once I have reached those goals *then* I introduce a simple breath-awareness activity. I call this Phase 2.

The breathing activity involves asking the children to breathe in and out of their noses while being aware of their tummies rising and falling in time with their breath. Keep it simple. Some children will get it quickly, some not so quickly. Be patient and persevere.

Our book *Frog's Breathtaking Speech* deals with the breathing element in greater depth. That said, you will notice that I have built breath awareness into the story, when Ladybird lands gently on Dog's tummy.

Take action – you'll be amazed

I hope you have found the idea of relaxation inspiring and do try Ladybird Relaxation with your class, children or child. You will be amazed by the results. If you would like any help or further information please get in touch at info@yogaatschool.org.uk or www.yogaatschool.org.uk.

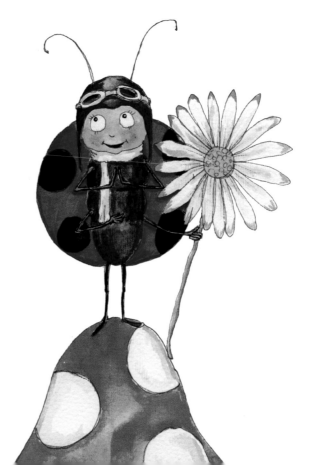

Ladybird's Remarkable Relaxation

Frog, Dog, Flamingo and Dragon paced anxiously around and around the Old Brown Tree.

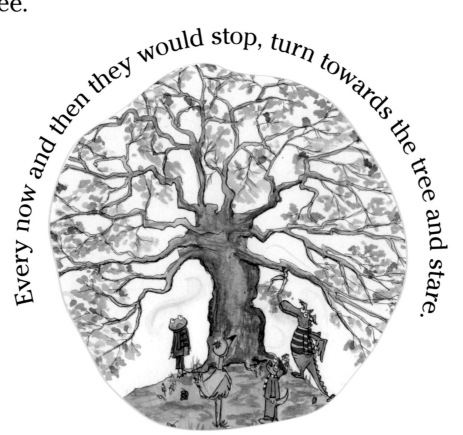

Every now and then they would stop, turn towards the tree and stare.

While quietly high above them sat Ladybird watching. Watching the sky, watching the wind, watching the clouds and, above all, watching the four friends pacing anxiously around the tree.

"What's the matter?" asked Ladybird politely as she landed softly on her favourite leaf. "You all look so worried."

"Well, if you must know," said Frog in the most miserable voice, "I have so much to do at home. There is so much to do that I don't know where to start."

Ladybird listened with interest and enquired, "Such as...?"

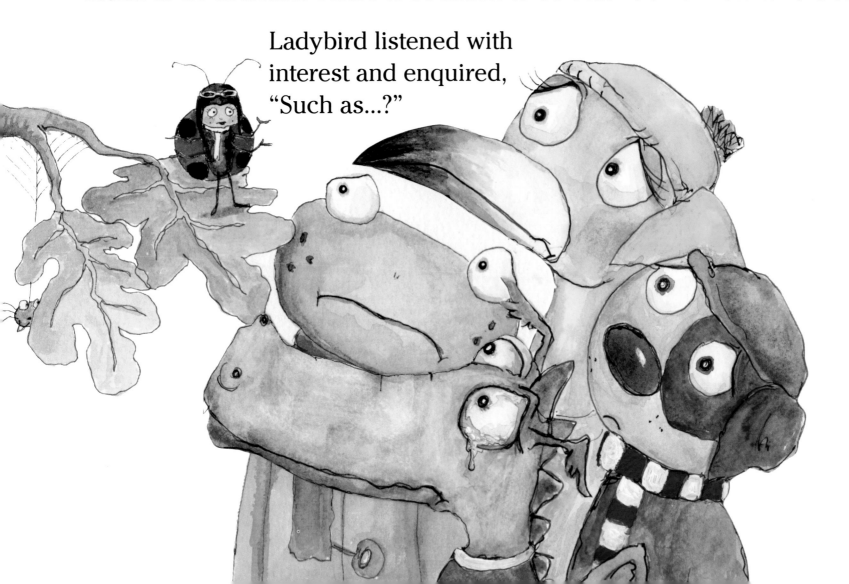

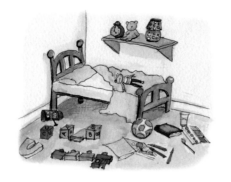 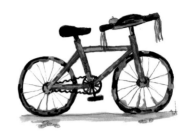

"Such as tidy my room. Such as clean my bike," listed Frog.

"Such as find the missing jigsaw piece that I hid from my dad. Such as help my sister with her maths homework."

"I see..." said Ladybird with an understanding voice.

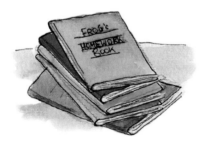

"And it's not just that. I have loads to do for school as well. It is," he continued, "all too much for me." As he spoke, a tiny tear ran down his cheek.

"And I," said Flamingo crossly, "I am so upset because I am called horrible names and laughed at in school, just because I am pink in places.

Sometimes I am pushed when we are lining up. But what really hurts is that they tell others not to play with me."

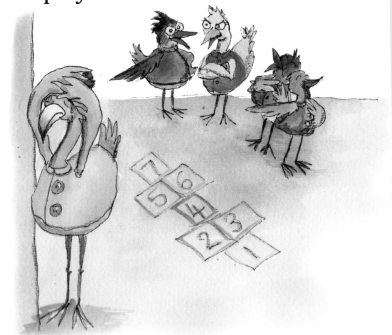

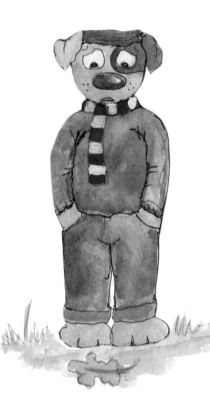

"And I," said Dog disappointedly, "I am upset because as hard as I try I cannot write stories. Not even the first line. Not even the first word."

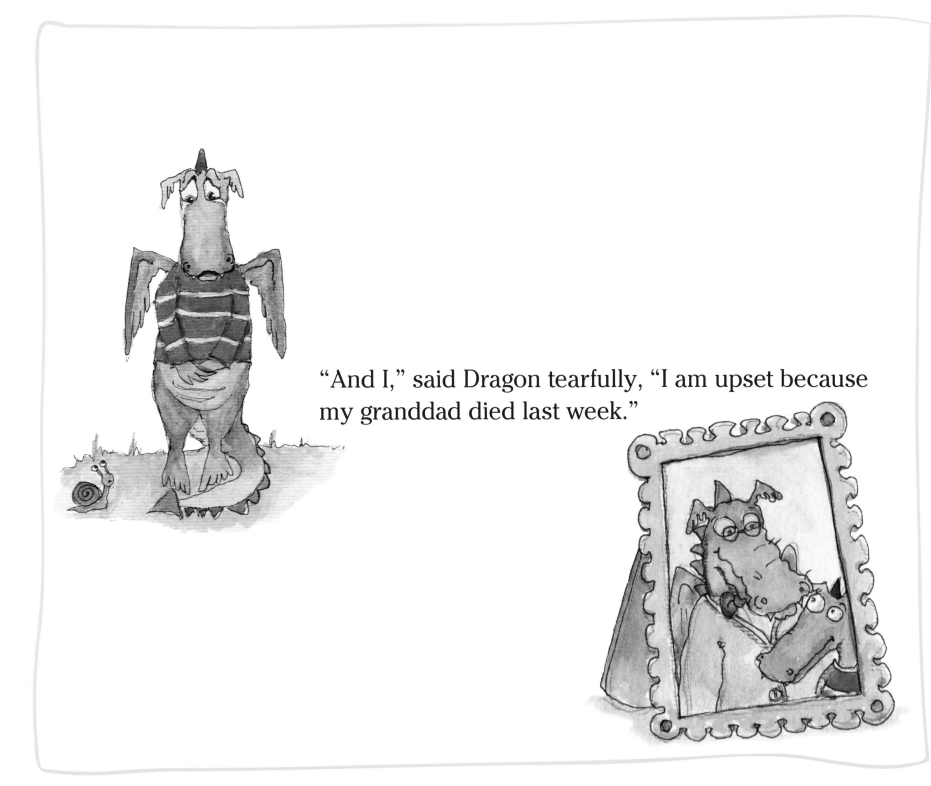

"And I," said Dragon tearfully, "I am upset because my granddad died last week."

Ladybird was silent for a few moments.

"I can help you all," she said suddenly.

"You mean," asked Frog hopefully, dabbing his cheek with a tissue, "that you will tidy my room, clean my bike, find the missing jigsaw piece and help my sister?"

"You mean," asked Flamingo hopefully, "that you will tell those bullies to stop pushing me and calling me pinkie-pooh, beaky and matchstick legs?"

"You mean," asked Dog timidly, "that you will write stories for me and let me say it's my work?"

"You mean," asked Dragon eagerly, accepting a tissue from Frog, "that you will magic my granddad alive?"

"No, Frog," replied Ladybird firmly and thoughtfully. "Cleaning your bike and all those tasks are for you to do. How would it help *you* if *I* did your jobs?"

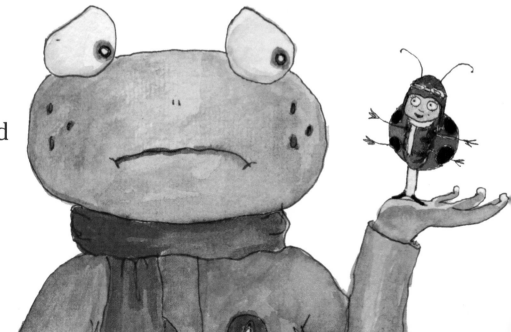

"No, Flamingo," said Ladybird firmly and warm-heartedly. "There are bullies everywhere. You have to learn to deal with bullies. How would it help *you* if *I* talked to them?"

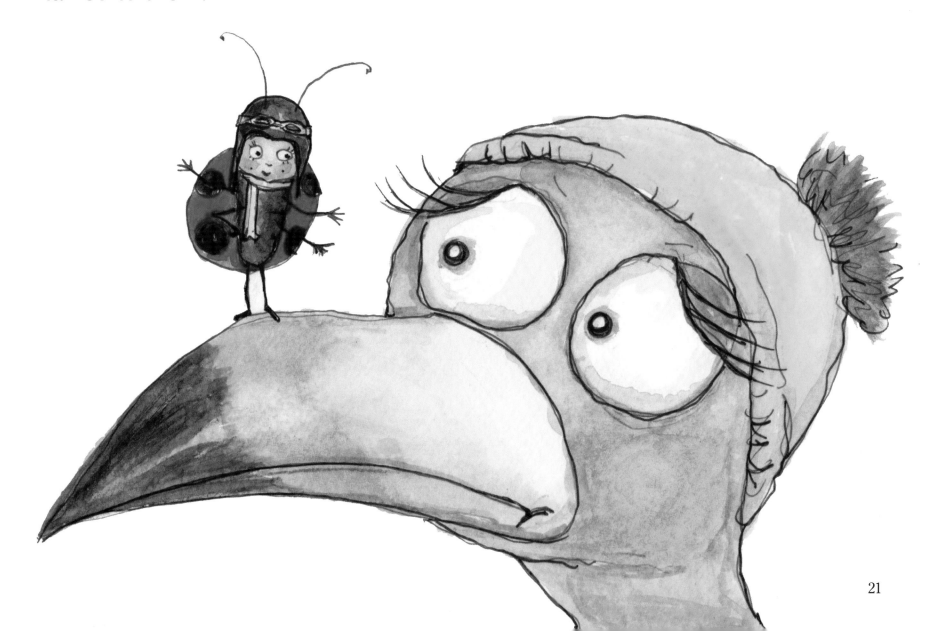

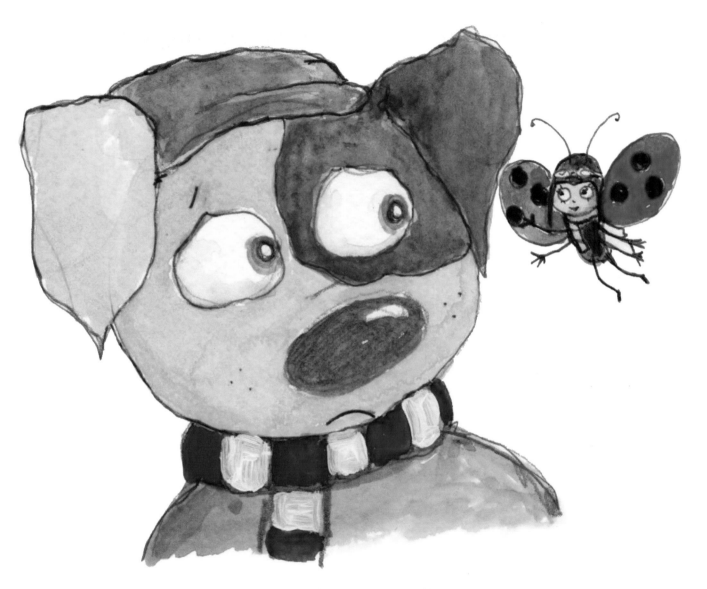

"No, Dog," said Ladybird firmly and affectionately. "You need to find the skills to write. How would it help *you* if *I* wrote your stories for you?"

"No, Dragon," said Ladybird firmly and caringly. "I cannot bring your granddad back, and I *cannot* stop you feeling upset and wanting to cry. But I *can* give you a precious gift to help you deal with the pain.

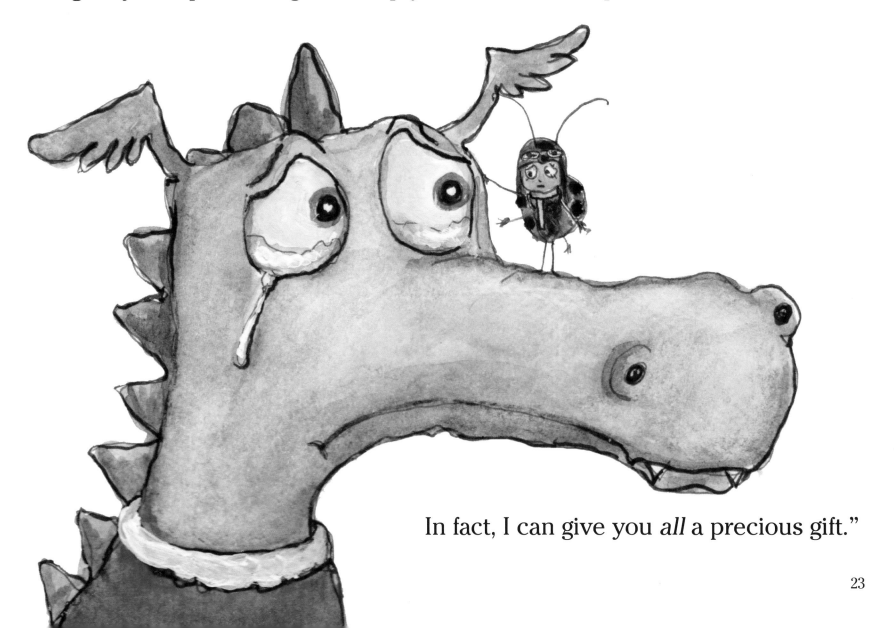

In fact, I can give you *all* a precious gift."

"A precious gift?" Frog, Flamingo, Dog and Dragon perked up.

"Is it a toy car?" enquired Frog.

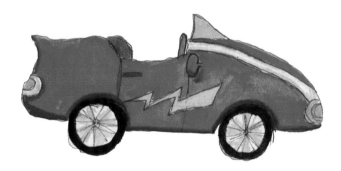

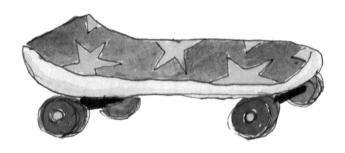

"A skateboard?" asked Dragon.

"A scooter?" suggested Dog.

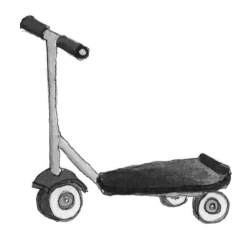

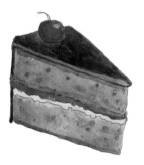

"Chocolate cake? I love chocolate cake. Is it chocolate cake?" pleaded Flamingo.

"No, it is none of those. Yes they are wonderful gifts; which, by the way, all cost money." Ladybird stopped talking as the four friends looked at each other, puzzled. "No," she continued, "the gift I will give you:

Costs not a penny   Can go any place   Weighs not a sausage   Takes up no space

Helps *you* respect *you*   Be brave, wise and strong

Ladybird's Remarkable Relaxation   Whatever comes along

This wonderful gift will help you deal with any problem that comes your way, including having too much on your plate, being bullied, feeling that you cannot succeed at something and helping you deal with sadness when someone dies or goes away."

Ladybird paused proudly, "I am going to teach you how to relax. I'm going to teach you Ladybird Relaxation."

"Oh crumbs," said Flamingo,
"I would rather have
chocolate cake."

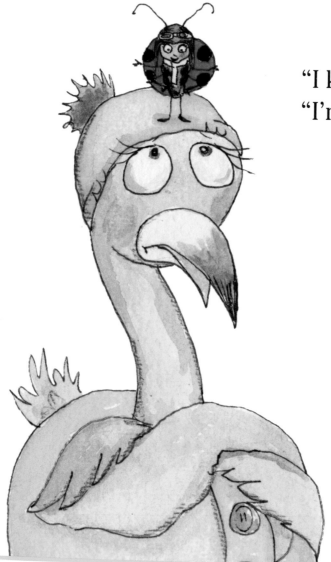

"I know," said Ladybird,
"I'm sure you would."

"I need a volunteer," said Ladybird. "Someone to help me teach you Ladybird Relaxation. Who is brave enough?"

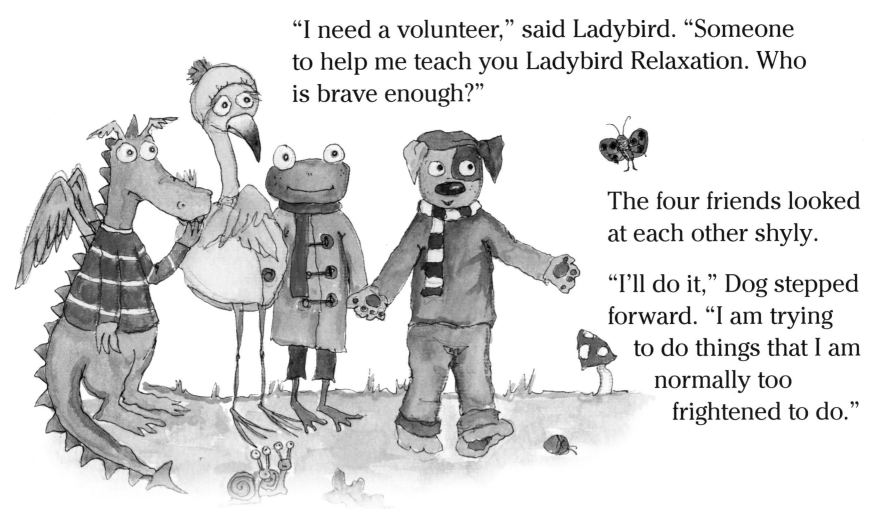

The four friends looked at each other shyly.

"I'll do it," Dog stepped forward. "I am trying to do things that I am normally too frightened to do."

"Well done, Dog, you are indeed very brave," said Ladybird.

Frog, Flamingo and Dragon watched curiously.

"If you look carefully in the roots of the tree you will find some purple mats that I keep so that folk can be comfortable in relaxation. Spread your mat on the grass and lie down quietly on your back with your arms by your sides. Have your palms facing towards the sky. Gently close your eyes and see if you can be aware of where on your body I am landing."

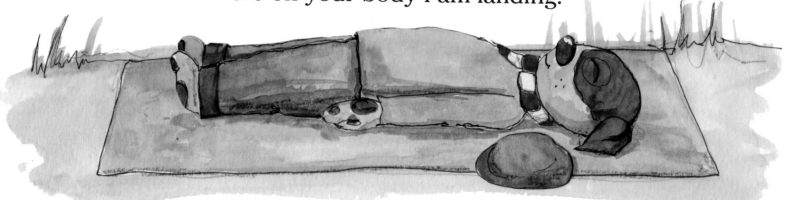

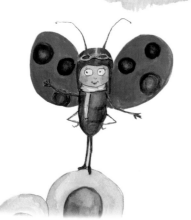

So saying, Ladybird flapped her wings, hovered above Dog and landed softly on his big toe. "Can you feel me?"

"Yes," whispered Dog, staying very still, "you're on my big toe."

Now Ladybird was tiny compared to Dog and his friends, so Dog had to concentrate *totally* to be aware of where Ladybird was landing.

Ladybird stayed there for about ten seconds, flapped her wings again, flew into the air above Dog, hovered for a moment and then landed smoothly on Dog's knee. *Which knee?* I hear you ask. Well, it was the knee that is on the same side as the big toe.

Another ten seconds passed. Ladybird flapped her wings again, flew into the air above Dog and then landed silkily on the tip of Dog's thumb. *Which thumb?* I hear you ask. Well, it was the thumb that is on the same side as the big toe and the knee.

After resting there for ten seconds, Ladybird flew into the air and then landed delicately on the tip of Dog's shoulder. *Which shoulder?* I hear you ask. It was the shoulder that is on the same side as the big toe, the knee and the thumb.

Ten seconds later and she flew into the air and landed featherly on the tip of Dog's nose. *Which nose?* I didn't hear anyone ask because Dogs only have ONE nose, just like you and me!

Ladybird stayed quietly on Dog's nose for another ten seconds, though it seemed like ages to Dog. Then she flew into the air and landed tenderly on the tip of Dog's shoulder. *Which shoulder?* I hear you ask. The *other* shoulder on the *other* side of Dog's body.

And so it continued.

Onto the *other* thumb, then... Onto the *other* knee, then... Onto the *other* big toe...

Each time she rested for about ten seconds before taking off again.

It may have been eleven or twelve seconds before Ladybird finally flapped her wings again, flew into the air above Dog and this time landed carefully on Dog's tummy.

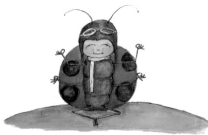

And there she stayed, still and serene.

As Frog, Flamingo and Dragon watched, they saw Ladybird slowly rising up and down. *Why is she rising up and down on Dog's tummy?* I hear you ask. The answer is...because Dog's tummy slowly rises up and down in time with his breathing, just like your tummy would if you were lying down on your back.

"This is the *best* bit," Ladybird whispered to Dog and his friends.

"Dog, I would like you to think about a problem you have. Ask yourself what *you* can do to solve that problem. Step back and look at the bigger picture. What action can you take? Take your time. If a plan comes into your mind, I want you to be determined to make it happen. If no plan comes up, don't worry, it may be hiding and pop up later. That often happens."

Ladybird fell silent.

Three long, calm, silent, peaceful minutes passed before she gracefully flapped her wings again and flew back to her favourite leaf on the tree.

Dog sat up slowly and opened his eyes.

"Do you know what?" he said. "I feel *so* relaxed. I rather like it."
     "Did you think about your problem, Dog?"
"Yes I did," replied Dog.
     "Did you think about a plan of action?"
"Yes I did," replied Dog.
     "And are you determined to make it happen?"
"I will do my best," replied Dog.

"Can we do it again, please?" asked Dog excitedly.

"Of course," replied Ladybird.
"Would you all like to have a go?"

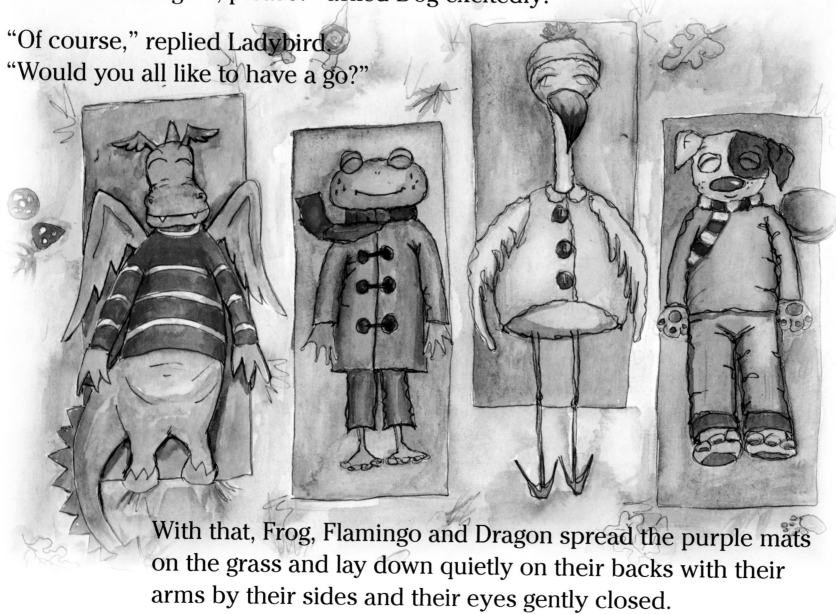

With that, Frog, Flamingo and Dragon spread the purple mats
on the grass and lay down quietly on their backs with their
arms by their sides and their eyes gently closed.

When Ladybird saw that the four friends were lying very still and quiet, she began the relaxation again. When they were all totally relaxed, she asked them to think about any problems they had, to see the bigger picture and, if a plan came up, to be determined to make it happen. Five minutes later the relaxation was complete.

Frog, Dog, Flamingo and Dragon sat up slowly, opened their eyes and looked around. Nothing was said. Everyone sat in silence, beaming from ear to ear.

Eventually Frog said, "Do you know what? I feel *so* relaxed. I rather like it too."

Dog, Flamingo and Dragon agreed.

Ladybird smiled. "Well done to you all, you were brilliant in relaxation. Do you think you can practise on your own?"

The four friends nodded enthusiastically.

"I must fly now," she said. "Do come and see me again. I will be very interested to hear how you are getting on."

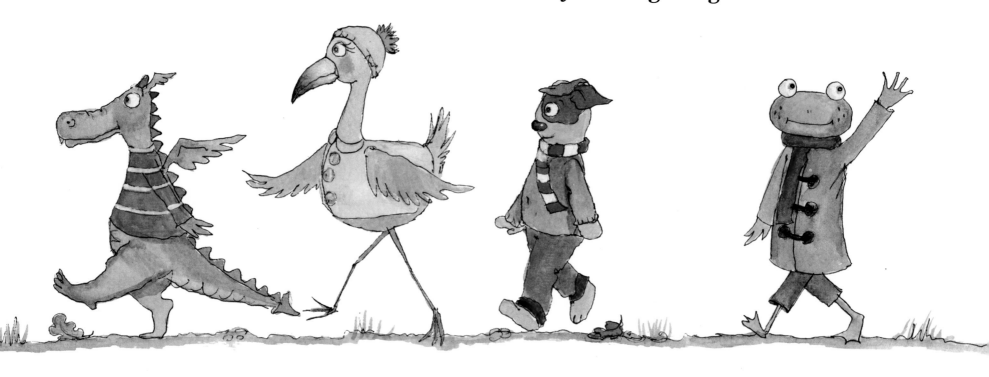

"Thank you, we will," they said as they skipped off along the path.

Three weeks just flew by. Frog, Dog, Flamingo and Dragon found themselves skipping cheerfully around and around the Old Brown Tree.

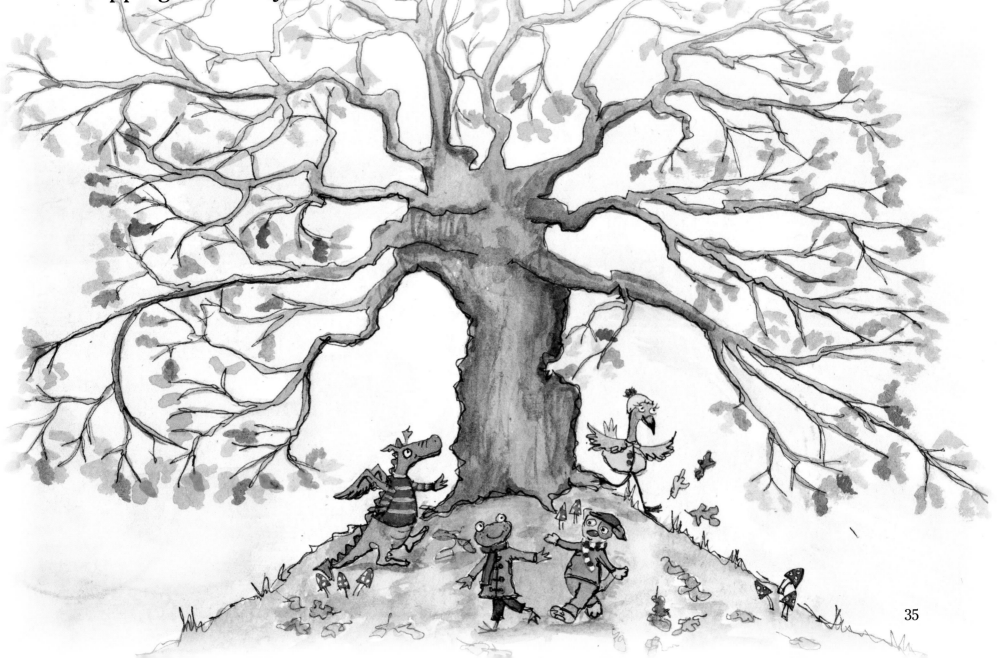

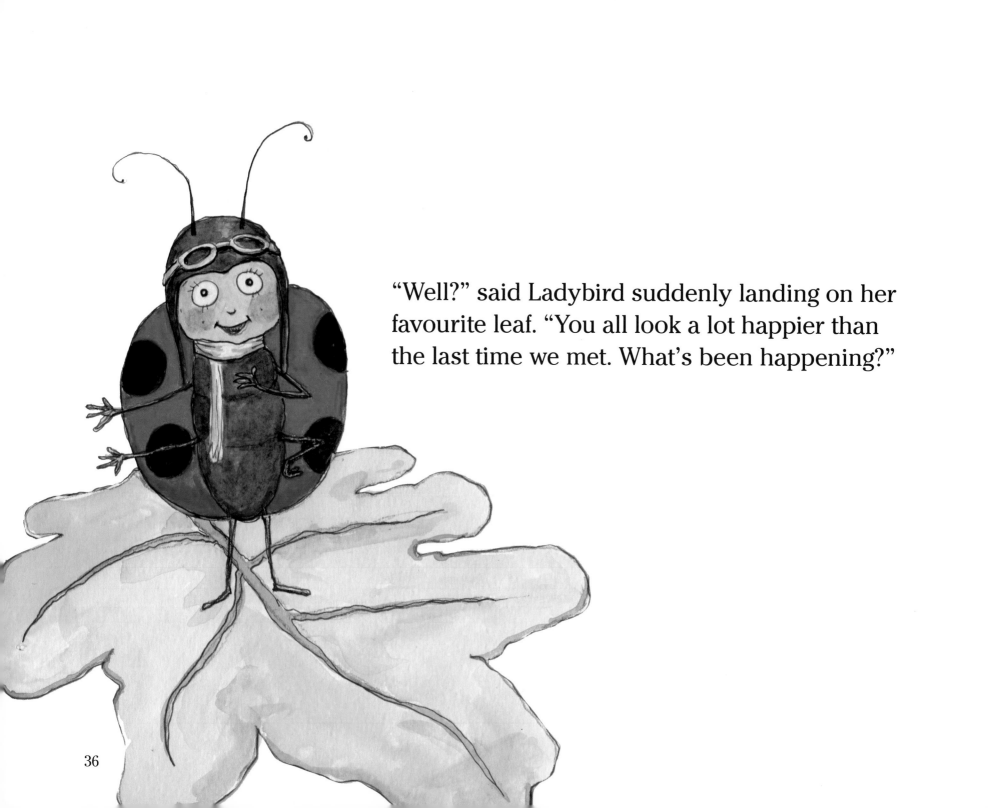

"Well?" said Ladybird suddenly landing on her favourite leaf. "You all look a lot happier than the last time we met. What's been happening?"

Frog stepped forward to tell his story.

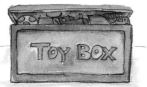

"During our relaxation I realised that it would take much less time to clear up my room. After all, it's only toys and things and they can go back in the toy box. I also realised that I love my bike! I was looking forward to riding round town with the clean chrome glistening in the sunshine, especially since I don't need stabilisers any more. I decided to clean my bike that *very* afternoon.

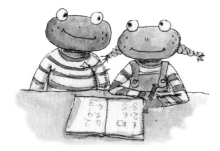

Then I remembered that my sister's pretty smart. I knew that I'd only need to show her a couple of times how to make numbers up to ten and then she'd get it – and she did.

Before relaxation my mind was like a tangle of string. Now it's like a short, straight, sharp arrow and I can see clearly what I need to do.

Thank you, Ladybird, thank you for your *remarkable* relaxation."

It was Flamingo's turn to step forward and tell her story.

"During relaxation I realised that I had to take action to deal with the bullies. When I arrived at school the next day I spotted the four bullies waiting in their corner of the playground. Already they were calling me names and laughing at me. This time I was ready. I gave my teacher the letter that I had written the night before, which told of the horrible things that the bullies had said and done. It was during relaxation that I decided not to put up with this behaviour and that I must respect myself more. My teacher read the letter, smiled and asked me what I planned to do next. So I told her:

'I want you to come with me because I want to speak to the bullies and I want you to be there to support me.'

We walked out into the playground and across to the bullies. Everyone was watching. I was scared, yet I was also determined. As I looked into their eyes I announced firmly:

'I want you to know that I will no longer put up with your bullying.' I paused, thinking to myself how brave I was. 'You can see that I have now told my teacher about all the things you have said and done, and she will take action.' My teacher nodded sternly in agreement.

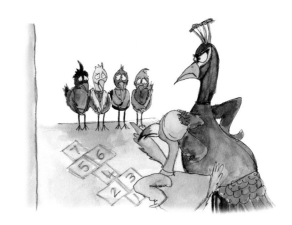

'No more will you bully me because I am pink, or have skinny legs or a long beak. We will also make sure that you do not bully *anyone* because of their colour or the way they look.' The bullies nodded quietly. It seemed they had no more to say.

Before relaxation I wanted to run away from school, run away from the bullies. Now I know exactly what to do. Be brave, tell my teacher and stand up for myself.

Thank you, Ladybird, thank you for your *remarkable* relaxation."

"How about you, Dog?" said Ladybird. "Did you take action about your writing problem?"

Dog stepped forward to tell his story.

"During relaxation I had a great plan and I was determined to put it into action. I asked Frog, Flamingo and Dragon to show me how *they* started stories and they each showed me a different way. On top of that I re-read my collection of favourite books to see how they started too. I could see how others did it and this gave me heaps of ideas. When I arrived at school three days later I was prepared.

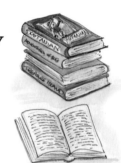

Before relaxation I was frightened to write anything because I thought it would be rubbish. Now I have a better idea of how to start a story. Now I know exactly what to do. Next I will learn how to end a story.

Thank you, Ladybird, thank you for your *remarkable* relaxation."

"Well, Dragon," said Ladybird, "you had a very difficult problem. Have you anything to tell us?"

Dragon stepped forward. For just a moment he could not speak.

"Take your time," Ladybird said.

Dragon began his story.

"During relaxation I couldn't think of any plans. I could only think how sad I was. A few days later I decided to talk to my mum and dad about it. They explained that it was normal to be sad because my granddad had died; that it was normal to cry; that they were sad too and were crying a lot. And, yes, I did cry a lot. Some days I felt better and some days I didn't. As time has passed I have found that I cry less and there are more days when I feel better.

Before relaxation I would never show my feelings. Now I know exactly what to do.

Thank you, Ladybird, thank you for your *remarkable* relaxation."

41

"You are all very welcome," said Ladybird. "I hope that you will tell others about this relaxation. Everyone experiences problems in their life. It is impossible to escape problems. So it is good to have a way to deal with them. Can you think of a way to tell others about it?"

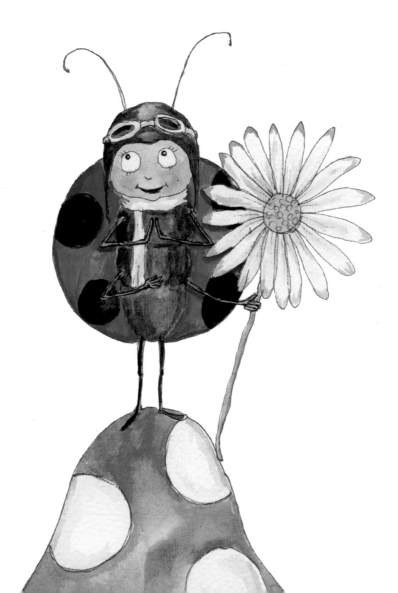

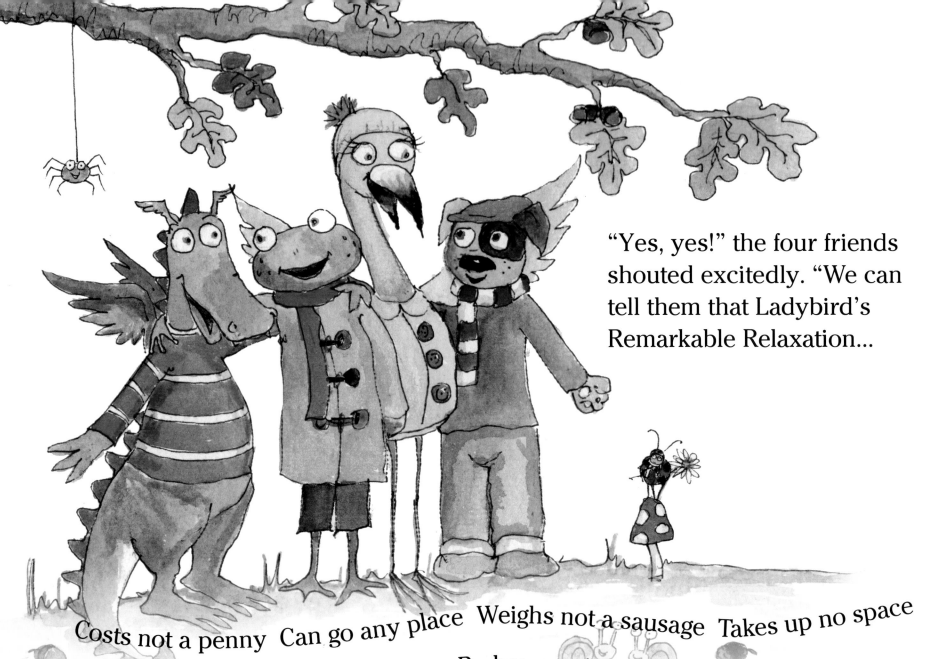

"Yes, yes!" the four friends shouted excitedly. "We can tell them that Ladybird's Remarkable Relaxation...

Costs not a penny Can go any place Weighs not a sausage Takes up no space

Helps *you* respect you Be brave, wise and strong

Ladybird's Remarkable Relaxation Whatever comes along."

43

"Well done, all of you," applauded Ladybird. "There's just one thing, Frog, that I am not clear about."

"What's that?" asked Frog, surprised.

"Did you find the missing piece to your dad's jigsaw puzzle?"

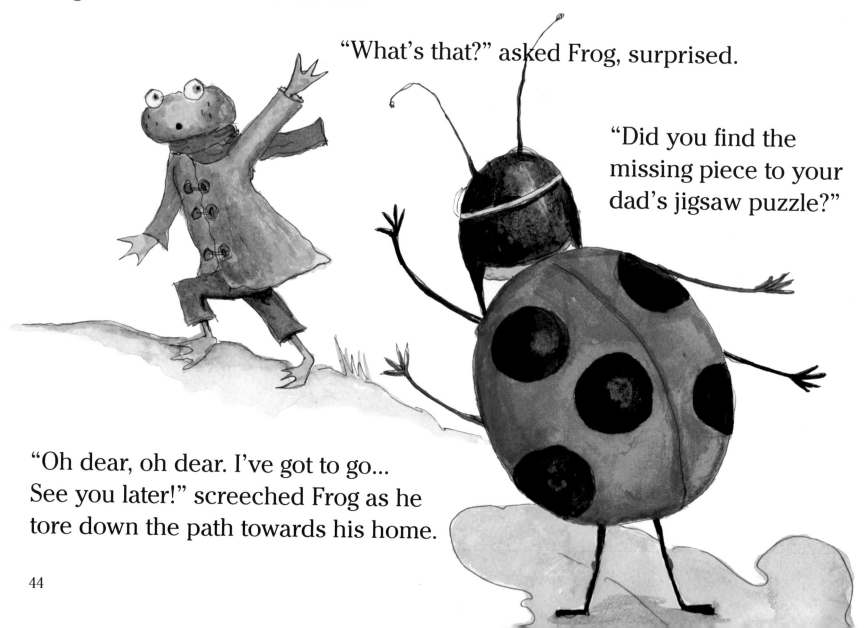

"Oh dear, oh dear. I've got to go... See you later!" screeched Frog as he tore down the path towards his home.

44

How to Teach Ladybird Relaxation

Ladybird Relaxation can be divided into three phases:

Phase 1 (week 1–3): Teaching, learning and reinforcement

This is the relaxation itself, without any breathing element or element of using the relaxation to deal with problems. Reinforce the technique as many times as possible over a three-week period. By the end of the period Ladybird Relaxation will be well ingrained.

Phase 2 (week 4 onwards): Introducing the breath element

Now is the time to bring in the breath element, and to include it in future relaxations.

QUICK REMINDER

The breathing activity involves asking the children to breathe in and out of their noses while being aware of their tummies rising and falling in time with their breath. Keep it simple. Some children will get it quickly, some not so quickly. Be patient and persevere.

Phase 3 (week 6 onwards): Introducing the element of dealing with problems

Towards the end of Ladybird Relaxation children will be most relaxed and therefore most receptive to the idea of looking at the bigger picture. You know best how to communicate this idea to your child or class.

Remind them about the part of the story when Ladybird asked Dog:

> "Dog, I would like you to think about a problem you have. Ask yourself what *you* can do to solve that problem. Step back and look at the bigger picture. What action can you take? Take your time. If a plan comes into your mind, I want you to be determined to make it happen. If no plan comes up, don't worry, it may be hiding and pop up later. That often happens."

Remind the children about Dog's problem and perhaps one of the other's. Remind them what action Dog took. Keep it short and to the point. Pace, as ever, is the key. Ask them to step back and look at the bigger picture and then relate it to a problem in their own lives. Ask what action they could take. How would that action involve using courage, wisdom and kindness?

Allow a minute or so for them to think about this, and then complete the relaxation before saying: "And then the ladybird flaps its wings and flies away, back to its home in the trees."

Finally, you could ask if anyone had an experience similar to Dog, Frog, Dragon or Flamingo. If anyone wants to talk about their experience, you may find it better to talk privately rather than in front of whole class. I am sure you will make sound judgements about that based on courage, wisdom and compassion.

Realistic outcomes

Please be realistic with your expectations for outcomes. On the one hand, some children will have had positive experiences and will be eager to share them. On the other, some may not. In addition there will be some who are at different places in between those two extremes. Each child will react in their own way. I am certain you will understand and respect that and ensure that whatever their experience you can genuinely tell them:

"That is fine… You are OK."

At the very best… At the very worst…

The way that I see it is this: at the very best that child is learning how to relax, see the bigger picture and deal with life; and at the very worst the child is learning how to relax… And, of course, have fun!

Enjoy!

Ladybird Relaxation Script

Set up

Have the children lie on mats on their backs with their arms by their sides, palms upwards. Make sure each child has enough space so as not to disturb anyone else. Allow the children time to settle and become comfortable. Ask the children to close their eyes gently. When everyone is ready proceed with Phase 1 using the script that follows. Please feel free to change it to match the needs of your child or your class.

The script

A tiny, shy, tired ladybird needs to find somewhere safe to rest for a while. She looks down and sees you lying so still and calmly. She thinks you look kind so she lands carefully on...
your **big toe**; and stays for a moment.

Then Ladybird flaps her wings and flies in the air and lands gently on...
your **knee**; and stays there for another moment.

Ladybird flaps her wings again, flies in the air and lands softly on...
the **tip of your thumb**; and stays there for a moment too.

Ladybird flaps her wings again, flies in the air and lands softly on...
your **shoulder**; happy to stay there for a moment.

Ladybird flaps her wings and flies in the air and this time lands gently on...

the **tip of your nose**; and stays there for a tiny moment, sharing your stillness.

Ladybird flaps her wings and flies in the air and lands softly on...
your ***other* shoulder**; and is so comfortable that she stays there for another moment.

Ladybird flaps her wings and flies in the air and lands carefully on...
your ***other* thumb**; she is so happy to share your calmness she stays there for a few moments more.

Ladybird flaps her wings and flies in the air and lands softly on...
your ***other* knee**; where she stays for just another moment, very still, like you.

Ladybird flaps her wings and flies in the air and lands carefully on...
your ***other* big toe**; and settles down quietly, calmly and happily.

This is the best bit. Allow the children to relax in silence for 1–2 minutes. Trust your judgement to bring them up when you think the time is right. Complete the relaxation by saying:

And then Ladybird flaps her wings and flies away, back to her home in the trees.

Allow and enjoy a few more moments of silence as the children re-orientate themselves.

ABOUT THE AUTHORS

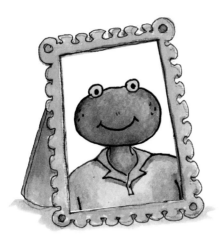

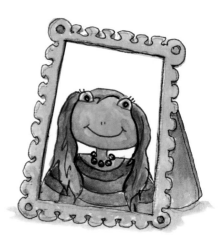

Michael Chissick has been teaching yoga to children in primary mainstream and special needs schools as part of the integrated school day since 1999. He is a leading specialist in teaching yoga to children with autistic spectrum disorders (ASD). Michael continues to train and mentor students who want to teach yoga to children, and is well known as "The Teachers' Teacher." Michael is acknowledged by the yoga community and the education sector as a genuine leader in this field.

Michael is happy to give advice and guidance about teaching and training to anyone involved in teaching yoga to children. Contact info@yogaatschool.org.uk or visit the website at www.yogaatschool.org.uk.

Sarah Peacock's delightful characterisation of Ladybird and her friends are typical examples of her unique talent. Her illustrations are detailed, fun, story enhancing and reflect the moods of each character. Following a first class degree in Theatre Design, Sarah then completed her teacher training in 2004. Her passion for art and illustration are in abundant evidence around the Hertfordshire primary school where she teaches; enhancing not only the school environment, but also providing inspiration to the children.

You can contact Sarah at sarahpeacock30@yahoo.co.uk.